DEMENTIA COOKBOOK FOR SENIORS

Healthy and Delicious recipes to regain memory loss and boost your brain function

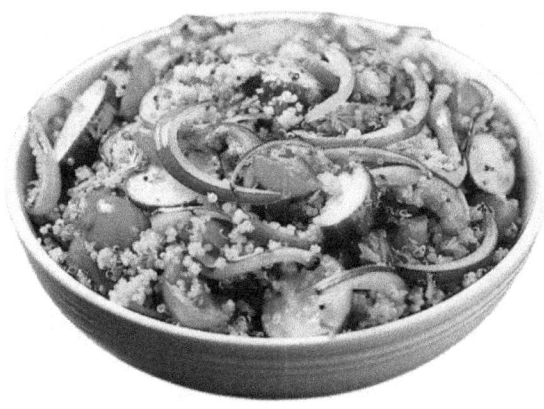

Dr. Malvin harison

TABLE OF CONTENT

Introduction

Welcome to "Mindful Cooking: A Dementia Cookbook for Seniors," a culinary journey crafted with care for those navigating the challenges of dementia. In these pages, we embark on a flavorful exploration, recognizing that the art of cooking can be a powerful ally in enhancing the well-being of both mind and body. Every recipe is thoughtfully designed to engage the senses, evoke memories, and provide nourishment tailored to the unique needs of seniors facing dementia.

Join us in this culinary odyssey, where the kitchen becomes a canvas for connection, joy, and the preservation of cherished moments. Let the aromas, textures, and tastes within these recipes create a symphony of sensory experiences, bringing comfort and delight to both the cook and the savored.

What is Dementia?

Dementia is not a specific disease but rather a term used to describe a decline in mental function, affecting memory, reasoning, language, coordination, mood, and behavior. It results from infections or diseases that impact areas of the brain involved in learning, memory, decision-making, or language. Alzheimer's disease is the most common cause of dementia, but other contributing factors include vascular dementia, dementia with Lewy bodies, frontotemporal dementia, mixed dementia, and dementia related to Parkinson's disease. Additionally, reversible conditions like medication side effects or thyroid problems can lead to dementia-like symptoms.

Dementia is prevalent in older individuals, with about 5% to 8% of people over the age of 65 experiencing some form of dementia. This prevalence doubles every five years beyond the age of 65. Approximately half of individuals aged 85 and older are estimated to have dementia. It is crucial to understand that dementia is an umbrella term encompassing various conditions, with Alzheimer's disease being the most frequently identified underlying cause.

Importance of a Proper Diet for Dementia Seniors

A well-balanced and nutritious diet plays a crucial role in supporting the overall health and well-being of seniors facing dementia. Here are key reasons highlighting the importance of a proper diet:

1. **Brain Health**: Certain nutrients, such as omega-3 fatty acids, antioxidants, and vitamins, are associated with cognitive function and brain health. A proper diet can contribute to maintaining and supporting cognitive abilities.

2. Energy and Nutrient Intake: Dementia can lead to challenges in eating and maintaining a healthy weight. A proper diet ensures an adequate intake of essential nutrients and energy, addressing nutritional needs and preventing malnutrition.

3. Physical Health: A nutritious diet supports overall physical health, helping to manage conditions that often accompany dementia, such as diabetes, heart disease, and high blood pressure.

4. Emotional Well-being: Nutrient-rich foods can positively influence mood and emotional well-being. A balanced diet may help reduce symptoms of depression and anxiety, common in individuals with dementia.

5. Enhanced Quality of Life: A well-planned diet can contribute to an improved quality of life for dementia seniors by addressing nutritional requirements and promoting overall health, potentially slowing down the progression of the condition.

Complications of an Inadequate Diet for Dementia Seniors

Not adhering to a proper diet can lead to various complications for seniors with dementia:

1. Malnutrition: Difficulty in eating, forgetting to eat, or changes in taste and smell can contribute to inadequate food intake, leading to malnutrition. Malnutrition can exacerbate cognitive decline and weaken the overall health of individuals with dementia.

2. Increased Risk of Infections: Poor nutrition weakens the immune system, making seniors more susceptible to infections. Dementia seniors may face challenges in maintaining proper hygiene and may require additional nutritional support to combat infections effectively.

3. Worsening Cognitive Function: Inadequate intake of essential nutrients can accelerate cognitive decline. The brain requires proper nourishment to function optimally, and a lack of key nutrients may contribute to a faster deterioration of cognitive abilities.

4. Muscle Weakness and Fatigue: Malnutrition can result in muscle weakness and fatigue, further reducing mobility and independence. This may contribute to a decline in overall physical health and increase the risk of falls and injuries.

5. Agitation and Behavioral Issues: Poor nutrition may contribute to increased agitation, aggression, or other behavioral issues in individuals with dementia. Meeting nutritional needs is essential for maintaining emotional well-being and managing behavioral symptoms.

Food to Include for Dementia Seniors

1. Fatty Fish: Rich in omega-3 fatty acids, fish like salmon and trout support brain health and cognitive function.

2. Berries: Blueberries, strawberries, and other berries are packed with antioxidants, which may help improve memory and cognitive function.

3. Leafy Greens: Spinach, kale, and other leafy greens are high in vitamins, minerals, and antioxidants that support overall health.

4. Nuts and Seeds: Almonds, walnuts, chia seeds, and flax seeds provide healthy fats, vitamins, and antioxidants beneficial for brain health.

5. Whole Grains: Brown rice, quinoa, and whole wheat provide a steady supply of energy and nutrients, promoting overall well-being.

6. Colorful Vegetables: Carrots, bell peppers, and sweet potatoes are rich in vitamins and antioxidants that support brain health.

7. Lean Proteins: Skinless poultry, lean beef, and plant-based proteins like beans and lentils contribute to muscle health and overall nutrition.

8. Low-Fat Dairy: Milk, yogurt, and cheese provide essential nutrients like calcium and vitamin D for bone health.

9. Healthy Fats: Olive oil, avocados, and coconut oil contain healthy fats that support brain function.

10. Herbs and Spices: Turmeric, cinnamon, and other herbs/spices have anti-inflammatory and antioxidant properties.

Foods to Limit or Avoid

1. Processed Foods: Minimize the consumption of processed foods high in salt, sugar, and unhealthy fats.

2. Sugary Snacks and Desserts: Reduce intake of candies, pastries, and sugary snacks, as excessive sugar may contribute to cognitive decline.

3. Saturated Fats: Limit the intake of red meat and full-fat dairy products, as high levels of saturated fats may negatively impact heart health.

4. Excessive Salt: Reduce salt intake to support cardiovascular health; opt for herbs and spices for flavoring instead.

5. Trans Fats: Avoid foods with trans fats, commonly found in some processed and fried foods.

6. Highly Processed Foods: Minimize the consumption of pre-packaged meals, as they often contain additives and preservatives.

7. Alcohol: Limit alcohol intake, as excessive alcohol can impair cognitive function and interact negatively with medications.

8. Caffeine: While moderate caffeine intake is generally safe, excessive consumption may lead to dehydration; ensure seniors stay hydrated.

9. Highly Caloric Foods: Be cautious with high-calorie foods that may contribute to weight gain and related health issues.

10. Individual Allergies or Sensitivities: Consider any specific allergies or sensitivities the individual may have and tailor the diet accordingly.

Chapter 1: Delicious Breakfast Recipes

Here are 10 nutrient-rich and dementia-friendly breakfast recipes that prioritize brain health.

1. Blueberry Oatmeal

Ingredients
- 1/2 cup old-fashioned oats
- 1 cup milk (dairy or plant-based)
- 1/2 cup fresh blueberries
- 1 tablespoon chia seeds
- 1 tablespoon honey

Instructions
1. Combine oats and milk in a saucepan over medium heat.
2. Cook until the oats are tender and the mixture thickens.
3. Stir in blueberries, chia seeds, and honey.
4. Cook for an additional 2 minutes.
5. Serve warm.

Nutritional Value (per serving)
- Calories: 300
- Protein: 8g
- Fiber: 7g
- Healthy Fats: 6g
Cooking Time: 10 minutes

2. Greek Yogurt Parfait

Ingredients
- 1/2 cup Greek yogurt
- 1/4 cup granola (low-sugar)
- 1/2 cup mixed berries (strawberries, blueberries)
- 1 tablespoon almond slices

Instructions
1. In a glass, turn Greek yogurt, granola, and mixed berries into layers.
2. Repeat the layers.
3. Top with almond slices.
4. Serve chilled.

Nutritional Value (per serving)
- Calories: 250
- Protein: 15g
- Fiber: 5g
- Healthy Fats: 8g

Cooking Time: 5 minutes

3. Spinach and Feta Omelette

Ingredients
- 2 eggs
- 1/2 cup fresh spinach (chopped)
- 2 tablespoons feta cheese (crumbled)
- 1/4 cup cherry tomatoes (halved)
- 1 teaspoon olive oil

Instructions
1. Whisk eggs in a bowl.
2. Heat olive oil in a non-stick pan.
3. Add spinach and cook until wilted.
4. Pour whisked eggs over spinach.
5. Sprinkle feta and tomatoes on top.
6. Cook until eggs are set.
7. Fold and serve.

Nutritional Value (per serving)
- Calories: 280
- Protein: 18g
- Fiber: 3g
- Healthy Fats: 20g

Cooking Time: 8 minutes

4. Chia Seed Pudding

Ingredients

- 2 tablespoons chia seeds
- 1/2 cup almond milk
- 1/2 teaspoon vanilla extract
- 1/4 cup mango chunks

Instructions

1. Mix chia seeds, almond milk, and vanilla extract in a bowl.
2. Refrigerate overnight or until a pudding-like consistency is achieved.
3. Top with mango chunks before serving.

Nutritional Value (per serving)

- Calories: 180
- Protein: 4g
- Fiber: 8g
- Healthy Fats: 8g

Cooking Time: Overnight (preparation time: 5 minutes)

5. Whole Grain Toast with Avocado

Ingredients
- 1 slice whole grain bread (toasted)
- 1/2 avocado (sliced)
- 1 teaspoon lemon juice
- Pinch of black pepper

Instructions
1. Toast the bread slice.
2. Spread sliced avocado on the toast.
3. Drizzle with lemon juice and sprinkle black pepper.
4. Serve immediately.

Nutritional Value (per serving)
- Calories: 200
- Protein: 4g
- Fiber: 6g
- Healthy Fats: 12g

Cooking Time: 5 minutes

6. Coconut-Berry Smoothie

Ingredients
- 1/2 cup coconut water
- 1/2 cup mixed berries (strawberries, blueberries)

- 1/2 banana
- 1 tablespoon coconut oil

Instructions

1. Blend coconut water, mixed berries, banana, and coconut oil until smooth.
2. Pour into a glass and serve.

Nutritional Value (per serving)

- Calories: 220
- Protein: 2g
- Fiber: 5g
- Healthy Fats: 14g

Cooking Time: 3 minutes

7. Sweet Potato Pancakes

Ingredients

- 1/2 cup cooked sweet potato (mashed)
- 2 eggs
- 1/4 teaspoon cinnamon
- 1 tablespoon maple syrup (optional)

Instructions

1. In a bowl, mix mashed sweet potato, eggs, and cinnamon.
2. Heat a pan and spoon batter to make small pancakes.

3. Cook until both sides are golden brown.

4. Drizzle with maple syrup if desired.

Nutritional Value (per serving)

- Calories: 230
- Protein: 9g
- Fiber: 3g
- Healthy Fats: 8g

Cooking Time: 10 minutes

8. Berry-Nut Breakfast Quinoa

Ingredients

- 1/2 cup cooked quinoa
- 1/4 cup almond milk
- 1/2 cup mixed berries (raspberries, blackberries)
- 1 tablespoon chopped walnuts

Instructions

1. Combine cooked quinoa and almond milk in a bowl.

2. Top with mixed berries and chopped walnuts.

3. Mix well and serve.

Nutritional Value (per serving)

- Calories: 220

- Protein: 8g
- Fiber: 6g
- Healthy Fats: 7g
Cooking Time: 5 minutes

9. Apple-Cinnamon Oat Muffins

Ingredients
- 1/2 cup rolled oats
- 1/2 cup applesauce
- 1 egg
- 1/2 teaspoon cinnamon
- 1/4 cup chopped apples

Instructions
1. Preheat the oven to 350°F (175°C).
2. Mix rolled oats, applesauce, egg, cinnamon, and chopped apples in a bowl.
3. Spoon the mixture into muffin cups.
4. Bake for 15-20 minutes until golden.

Nutritional Value (per serving)
- Calories: 180
- Protein: 5g
- Fiber: 4g
- Healthy Fats: 3g
Cooking Time: 20 minutes

10. Mango-Coconut Chia Smoothie Bowl

Ingredients
- 1/2 cup mango chunks
- 1/2 cup coconut milk
- 2 tablespoons chia seeds

Toppings: Sliced bananas, shredded coconut

Instructions

1. Blend mango chunks, coconut milk, and chia seeds until smooth.

2. Pour into a bowl and add sliced bananas and shredded coconut on top.

3. Serve immediately.

Nutritional Value (per serving)
- Calories: 250
- Protein: 5g
- Fiber: 8g
- Healthy Fats: 15g

Cooking Time: 5 minutes

Chapter 2: Satisfying Lunch

Here are 10 nutrient-rich and dementia-friendly lunch recipes that prioritize brain health.

1. Salmon and Vegetable Stir-Fry

Ingredients

1. 6 oz salmon filet
2. 1 cup broccoli florets
3. 1 bell pepper, thinly sliced
4. 1 tablespoon olive oil
5. 2 cloves garlic, minced
6. 1 tablespoon low-sodium soy sauce

Instructions

1. Cut salmon into cubes.
2. Heat olive oil in a pan, add salmon, garlic, and stir.
3. Add broccoli and bell pepper, stir-fry until vegetables are tender.
4. Drizzle with soy sauce.
5. Serve over brown rice or quinoa.

Nutritional Value (per serving)
- Calories: 350
- Protein: 30g
- Fiber: 5g
- Healthy Fats: 15g

Cooking Time: 15 minutes

2. Quinoa and Vegetable Stuffed Peppers

Ingredients
1. 2 bell peppers, halved
2. 1 cup cooked quinoa
3. 1/2 cup black beans, washed and rinsed
4. 1/2 cup corn kernels
5. 1/4 cup diced tomatoes
6. 1/4 cup shredded cheese (optional)

Instructions
1. Preheat the oven to 375°F (190°C).
2. Mix cooked quinoa, black beans, corn, and diced tomatoes.
3. Stuff peppers with the mixture.
4. Top with shredded cheese if desired.
5. Bake for 20-25 minutes.

Nutritional Value (per serving)

- Calories: 280
- Protein: 12g
- Fiber: 8g
- Healthy Fats: 5g
Cooking Time: 25 minutes

3. Chicken and Vegetable Brown Rice Bowl

Ingredients
1. 4 oz grilled chicken breast, sliced
2. 1 cup cooked brown rice
3. 1 cup of mixed vegetables (carrots, peas, corn)
4. 1 tablespoon sesame oil
5. 2 green onions, chopped
6. 1 teaspoon low-sodium soy sauce

Instructions
1. Heat sesame oil in a pan, add mixed vegetables and stir.
2. Add sliced grilled chicken.
3. Stir in cooked brown rice.
4. Drizzle with soy sauce and garnish with chopped green onions.
5. Serve warm.

Nutritional Value (per serving)

- Calories: 400
- Protein: 25g
- Fiber: 6g
- Healthy Fats: 10g
Cooking Time: 20 minutes

4. Mediterranean Chickpea Salad

Ingredient

1. 1 can chickpeas, drained and rinsed
2. 1 cup cherry tomatoes, halved
3. 1 cucumber, diced
4. 1/4 cup feta cheese, crumbled
5. 2 tablespoons olive oil
6. 1 tablespoon balsamic vinegar

Instructions

1. Combine chickpeas, cherry tomatoes, cucumber, and feta cheese.
2. Spray with olive oil and balsamic vinegar.
3. Toss gently and refrigerate for 30 minutes.
4. Serve chilled.

Nutritional Value (per serving)

- Calories: 320

- Protein: 15g
- Fiber: 10g
- Healthy Fats: 12g

Cooking Time: 10 minutes (plus refrigeration time)

5. Vegetarian Lentil Soup

Ingredients

1. 1 cup dry green lentils, rinsed
2. 1 onion, diced
3. 2 carrots, sliced
4. 2 celery stalks, chopped
5. 3 cloves garlic, minced
6. 4 cups vegetable broth

Instructions

1. In a pot, sauté onion, carrots, celery, and garlic.
2. Add lentils and vegetable broth.
3. Let it boil, then leave it to seat for 30 minutes.
4. Season with herbs and spices as desired.
5. Serve hot.

Nutritional Value (per serving)

- Calories: 250

- Protein: 18g
- Fiber: 12g
- Healthy Fats: 2g
Cooking Time: 40 minutes

6. Sweet Potato and Chickpea Buddha Bowl

Ingredients
1. 1 medium sweet potato, cubed
2. 1 can chickpeas, drained and rinsed
3. 1 cup quinoa, cooked
4. 1 cup kale, chopped
5. 2 tablespoons tahini dressing

Instructions
1. Roast sweet potato cubes and chickpeas in the oven.
2. Arrange cooked quinoa, roasted sweet potatoes, chickpeas, and kale in a bowl.
3. Drizzle with tahini dressing.
4. Serve warm.

Nutritional Value (per serving)
- Calories: 380
- Protein: 15g
- Fiber: 12g
- Healthy Fats: 10g

Cooking Time: 30 minutes

7. Tomato Basil Avocado Sandwich

Ingredients
1. 2 slices whole-grain bread
2. 1 medium tomato, sliced
3. 1/2 avocado, mashed
4. Fresh basil leaves
5. Salt and pepper to taste

Instructions
1. Toast the whole-grain bread slices.
2. Spread mashed avocado on one slice.
3. Layer with tomato slices and fresh basil.
4. Sprinkle it with salt and pepper.
5. Add the other slice of bread as topping.

Nutritional Value (per serving)
- Calories: 280
- Protein: 7g
- Fiber: 8g
- Healthy Fats: 15g

Cooking Time: 5 minutes

8. Shrimp and Quinoa Salad

Ingredients

1. 8 oz shrimp, peeled and deveined
2. 1 cup cooked quinoa
3. 1 cup of mixed greens
4. 1/2 cup cherry tomatoes, halved
5. 1/4 cup feta cheese, crumbled
6. 1 tablespoon olive oil
7. 1 tablespoon lemon juice

Instructions

1. Sauté shrimp in olive oil until cooked.
2. In a bowl, combine cooked quinoa, mixed greens, cherry tomatoes, and feta cheese.
3. Top with sautéed shrimp.
4. Drizzle with lemon juice.
5. Serve chilled.

Nutritional Value (per serving)

- Calories: 320
- Protein: 25g
- Fiber: 5g
- Healthy Fats: 12g

Cooking Time: 15 minutes

9. Egg and Vegetable Wrap

Ingredients

1. 2 eggs, beaten
2. 1 whole-grain tortilla
3. 1/2 cup bell peppers, sliced
4. 1/4 cup black beans, washed and rinsed
5. 2 tablespoons salsa

Instructions

1. Scramble eggs in a pan until cooked.
2. Heat tortilla and place scrambled eggs on it.
3. Add diced bell peppers, black beans, and salsa.
4. Fold into a wrap and serve.

Nutritional Value (per serving)

- Calories: 280
- Protein: 15g
- Fiber: 8g
- Healthy Fats: 10g

Cooking Time: 10 minutes

10. Turkey and Vegetable Skewers

Ingredients

1. 8 oz turkey breast, cut into cubes
2. 1 zucchini, sliced
3. 1 red onion, sliced
4. Cherry tomatoes
5. 1 tablespoon olive oil
6. Herbs and spices for seasoning

Instructions

1. Season turkey cubes with herbs and spices.
2. Thread turkey, zucchini, red onion, and cherry tomatoes onto skewers.
3. Grill or bake until turkey is cooked through.
4. Drizzle with olive oil before serving.

Nutritional Value (per serving)

- Calories: 300
- Protein: 30g
- Fiber: 6g
- Healthy Fats: 8g

Cooking Time: 20 minutes

Chapter 3: Breathtaking dinner recipes

Here are 10 nutrient-rich and dementia-friendly dinner recipes that prioritize brain health.

1. Baked Salmon with Lemon and Herbs

Ingredients

1. 2 salmon filets
2. 1 lemon, sliced
3. 1 tablespoon olive oil
4. Fresh dill and rosemary
5. Salt and pepper to taste

Instructions

1. Preheat the oven to 375°F (190°C).
2. Place salmon filets on a baking sheet.
3. Spray with olive oil and add salt and pepper.
4. Top with lemon slices, dill, and rosemary.
5. Bake for 15-20 minutes.

Nutritional Value (per serving)

- Calories: 300
- Protein: 25g
- Healthy Fats: 18g
Cooking Time: 20 minutes

2. Vegetable Stir-Fry with Tofu

Ingredients

1. 1 cup tofu, cubed
2. 2 cups of mixed vegetables (broccoli, bell peppers, snap peas)
3. 2 tablespoons low-sodium soy sauce
4. 1 tablespoon sesame oil
5. 1 garlic clove, minced
6. Brown rice (optional)

Instructions

1. Leave tofu in sesame oil until slightly brown.
2. Add mixed vegetables and garlic, stir-fry until tender.
3. Spout soy sauce over the content and toss.
4. Serve alone or over brown rice.

Nutritional Value (per serving)

- Calories: 250
- Protein: 15g

- Healthy Fats: 12g
Cooking Time: 15 minutes

3. Quinoa Black Bean

Ingredients

1. 4 bell peppers, halved
2. 1 cup cooked quinoa
3. 1 can black beans, drained and rinsed
4. 1 cup corn kernels
5. 1/2 cup salsa
6. Shredded cheese (optional)

Instructions

1. Preheat the oven to 375°F (190°C).
2. Mix quinoa, black beans, corn, and salsa.
3. Stuff bell peppers with the mixture.
4. Top with shredded cheese if desired.
5. Bake for 20-25 minutes.

Nutritional Value (per serving)

- Calories: 280
- Protein: 12g
- Fiber: 8g
- Healthy Fats: 5g

Cooking Time: 25 minutes

4. Herb-Roasted Chicken with Vegetables

Ingredients

1. 4 chicken thighs
2. 1 lb baby potatoes, halved
3. 1 cup baby carrots
4. 2 tablespoons olive oil
5. Fresh thyme and rosemary
6. Salt and pepper to taste

Instructions

1. Preheat the oven to 400°F (200°C).
2. Toss chicken, potatoes, and carrots with olive oil.
3. Season with salt, pepper, thyme, and rosemary.
4. Roast for 30-35 minutes until chicken is cooked through.

Nutritional Value (per serving)

- Calories: 350
- Protein: 25g
- Healthy Fats: 15g

Cooking Time: 35 minutes

5. Mushroom and Spinach Quiche

Ingredients

1. 1 premade whole-grain pie crust
2. 1 cup mushrooms, sliced
3. 2 cups fresh spinach
4. 4 eggs
5. 1 cup milk (dairy or plant-based)
6. 1/2 cup shredded cheese (optional)

Instructions

1. Preheat the oven to 375°F (190°C).
2. Sauté mushrooms and spinach until wilted.
3. Whisk milk and egg together in a bowl.
4. Pour egg mixture into the pie crust.
5. Add sautéed mushrooms and spinach.
6. Top with shredded cheese if desired.
7. Bake for 30-35 minutes.

Nutritional Value (per serving)

- Calories: 280
- Protein: 14g
- Healthy Fats: 15g

Cooking Time: 35 minutes

6. Turkey and Vegetable Skillet

Ingredients

1. 1 lb ground turkey
2. 1 onion, diced
3. 2 bell peppers, sliced
4. 1 zucchini, diced
5. 1 can (15 oz) diced tomatoes
6. 1 teaspoon Italian seasoning

Instructions

1. In a skillet, cook ground turkey until browned.
2. Add diced onion, bell peppers, and zucchini.
3. Stir in diced tomatoes and Italian seasoning.
4. Simmer for 15-20 minutes.

Nutritional Value (per serving)

- Calories: 320
- Protein: 22g
- Healthy Fats: 10g

Cooking Time: 20 minutes

7. Salmon and Quinoa Salad

Ingredients

1. 2 salmon filets
2. 1 cup cooked quinoa
3. 1 cup cherry tomatoes, halved
4. 1 cucumber, diced
5. 1/4 cup feta cheese, crumbled
6. 2 tablespoons olive oil
7. 1 tablespoon balsamic vinegar

Instructions

1. Grill or bake salmon until cooked.
2. In a bowl, combine quinoa, cherry tomatoes, cucumber, and feta cheese.
3. Top with cooked salmon.
4. Sprinkle it with olive oil and balsamic vinegar.

Nutritional Value (per serving)

- Calories: 350
- Protein: 25g
- Healthy Fats: 18g

Cooking Time: 20 minutes

8. Vegetarian Lentil Curry

Ingredients

1. 1 cup dry green lentils, rinsed
2. 1 onion, diced
3. 2 carrots, sliced
4. 1 can (15 oz) diced tomatoes
5. 1 can (15 oz) coconut milk
6. 2 tablespoons curry powder

Instructions

1. In a pot, sauté onion until translucent.
2. Add lentils, carrots, diced tomatoes, coconut milk, and curry powder.
3. Simmer for 25-30 minutes.

Nutritional Value (per serving)

- Calories: 300
- Protein: 18g
- Healthy Fats: 12g

Cooking Time: 30 minutes

9. Eggplant and Chickpea Tagine

Ingredients

1. 1 large eggplant, diced
2. 1 can chickpeas, drained and rinsed
3. 1 onion, chopped

4. 2 cloves garlic, minced

5. 1 can (15 oz) crushed tomatoes

6. 1 teaspoon cumin

7. 1 teaspoon paprika

Instructions

1. Sauté onion and garlic until softened.

2. Add diced eggplant, chickpeas, crushed tomatoes, cumin, and paprika.

3. Simmer for 20-25 minutes.

Nutritional Value (per serving)

- Calories: 280

- Protein: 14g

- Healthy Fats: 10g

Cooking Time: 25 minutes

10. Lemon Garlic Shrimp with Whole Wheat Pasta

Ingredients

1. 8 oz whole wheat pasta

2. 8 oz shrimp, peeled and deveined

3. 2 tablespoons olive oil

4. 3 cloves garlic, minced

5. 1 lemon, juiced

6. Fresh parsley, chopped

Instructions

1. Cook whole wheat pasta according to package instructions.

2. In a pan, sauté shrimp in olive oil and minced garlic.

3. Add cooked pasta to the pan.

4. Squeeze lemon juice over the mixture.

5. Garnish with fresh parsley before serving.

Nutritional Value (per serving)

- Calories: 320
- Protein: 18g
- Healthy Fats: 10g

Cooking Time: 15 minutes

Chapter 4: Easy made Snacks and Dessert

Here are 10 nutrient-rich and dementia-friendly snack and dessert recipes that prioritize brain health.

1. Nutty Fruit Yogurt Parfait

Ingredients

1. 1 cup Greek yogurt
2. 1/4 cup of mixed nuts (almonds, walnuts)
3. 1/2 cup of mixed berries (blueberries, strawberries)
4. 1 tablespoon honey

Instructions

1. In a glass, layer Greek yogurt, mixed nuts, and berries.
2. Drizzle with honey.
3. Repeat layers.
4. Serve chilled.

Nutritional Value (per serving)

- Calories: 250

- Protein: 15g
- Healthy Fats: 12g
Preparation Time: 5 minutes

2. Apple Almond Butter

Ingredients
1. 1 medium apple, sliced
2. 2 tablespoons almond butter
3. Cinnamon for sprinkling

Instructions
1. Spread almond butter on apple slices.
2. Sprinkle with cinnamon.
3. Serve as a snack.

Nutritional Value (per serving)
- Calories: 180
- Protein: 4g
- Healthy Fats: 10g
Preparation Time: 5 minutes

3. Chia Pudding

Ingredients
1. 2 tablespoons chia seeds
2. 1 cup almond milk
3. 1/2 teaspoon vanilla extract

4. 1 tablespoon maple syrup

5. Fresh fruit for topping

Instructions

1. Combine chia seeds, almond milk, vanilla extract, and maple syrup.

2. Refrigerate for at least 2 hours or overnight.

3. Top with fresh fruit before serving.

Nutritional Value (per serving)

- Calories: 180
- Protein: 5g
- Healthy Fats: 8g

Preparation Time: 5 minutes (plus refrigeration time)

4. Vegetable Sticks with Hummus

Ingredients

1. Carrot and cucumber sticks

2. 1/4 cup hummus

Instructions

1. Arrange vegetable sticks on a plate.

2. Serve with hummus for dipping.

Nutritional Value (per serving)

- Calories: 120
- Protein: 4g

- Healthy Fats: 6g
Preparation Time: 5 minutes

5. Trail Mix

Ingredients
1. 1/2 cup almonds
2. 1/2 cup walnuts
3. 1/4 cup dark chocolate chips
4. 1/4 cup dried berries (cranberries, blueberries)

Instructions
1. Mix all ingredients in a bowl.
2. Portion into snack-sized bags.

Nutritional Value (per serving)
- Calories: 200
- Protein: 5g
- Healthy Fats: 12g
Preparation Time: 5 minutes

6. Berry and Yogurt Popsicles

Ingredients
1. 1 cup of mixed berries (strawberries, blueberries)
2. 1 cup Greek yogurt

3. 1 tablespoon honey

Instructions

1. Blend berries, Greek yogurt, and honey.
2. Pour into popsicle molds.
3. Freeze for at least 4 hours.

Nutritional Value (per serving)

- Calories: 120
- Protein: 6g
- Healthy Fats: 3g

Preparation Time: 10 minutes (plus freezing time)

7. Frozen Banana Bites

Ingredients

1. 2 bananas, sliced
2. 1/4 cup peanut butter
3. Dark chocolate for drizzling

Instructions

1. Spread peanut butter on banana slices.
2. Create banana sandwiches.
3. Drizzle with melted dark chocolate.
4. Freeze until solid.

Nutritional Value (per serving)

- Calories: 160
- Protein: 3g
- Healthy Fats: 8g

Preparation Time: 15 minutes (plus freezing time)

8. Avocado Chocolate Mousse

Ingredients

1. 2 ripe avocados
2. 1/4 cup cocoa powder
3. 1/4 cup maple syrup
4. 1/2 teaspoon vanilla extract

Instructions

1. Blend avocados, cocoa powder, maple syrup, and vanilla extract until smooth.
2. Refrigerate for 2 hours.
3. Serve chilled.

Nutritional Value (per serving)

- Calories: 180
- Protein: 3g
- Healthy Fats: 12g

Preparation Time: 10 minutes (plus refrigeration time)

9. Oatmeal Raisin Energy Bites

Ingredients

1. 1 cup rolled oats
2. 1/2 cup almond butter
3. 1/4 cup honey
4. 1/4 cup raisins
5. 1/2 teaspoon cinnamon

Instructions

1. Mix all ingredients in a bowl.
2. Roll into bite-sized balls.
3. Refrigerate for 1 hour.

Nutritional Value (per serving)

- Calories: 160
- Protein: 4g
- Healthy Fats: 8g

Preparation Time: 10 minutes (plus refrigeration time)

10. Coconut Mango Sorbet

Ingredients

1. 2 cups frozen mango chunks
2. 1/2 cup coconut milk
3. 1 tablespoon lime juice
4. Shredded coconut for topping

Instructions

1. Blend frozen mango, coconut milk, and lime juice until smooth.

2. Freeze for 2 hours.

3. Top with shredded coconut before serving.

Nutritional Value (per serving)

- Calories: 120
- Protein: 2g
- Healthy Fats: 5g

Preparation Time: 10 minutes (plus freezing time)

Chapter 5:Bonus 1

7- days Sample Meal Plan

Here's a 7-day meal plan for dementia management.

Day 1

Breakfast: Greek Yogurt Parfait
Lunch: Quinoa Black Bean
Dinner: Baked Salmon with Lemon and Herbs

Day 2

Breakfast: Chia Seed Pudding
Lunch: Vegetable Stir-Fry with Tofu
Dinner: Mushroom and Spinach Quiche

Day 3

Breakfast: Nutty Fruit Yogurt Parfait
Lunch: Lentil Curry with Vegetables
Dinner: Herb-Roasted Chicken with Vegetables

Day 4

Breakfast: Apple Slices with Almond Butter
Lunch: Turkey and Vegetable Skillet
Dinner: Salmon and Quinoa Salad

Day 5

Breakfast: Vegetable Sticks with Hummus
Lunch: Eggplant and Chickpea Tagine
Dinner: Lemon Garlic Shrimp with Whole Wheat Pasta

Day 6

Breakfast: Homemade Trail Mix
Lunch: Chicken Spinach Avocado Salad
Dinner: Sweet Potato and Black Bean Quesadillas

Day 7

Breakfast: Oatmeal Raisin Energy Bites

Lunch: Caprese Salad with Balsamic Glaze

Dinner: Grilled Vegetable and Chickpea Wrap

Chapter 6: Bonus 2

20 Juicing and Smoothie Recipes

Here are 20 juicing and smoothie recipes designed for dementia seniors.

1. Brain Boost Juice

Ingredients: Blueberries, spinach, kale, cucumber, and apple.
Instructions: Juice all ingredients and serve immediately.

2. Citrus Bliss

Ingredients: Oranges, grapefruit, carrots, and ginger.
Instructions: Juice citrus fruits and carrots, add a touch of ginger, and serve.

3. Green Elixir

Ingredients: Celery, cucumber, kale, green apple, and lemon.

Instructions: Juice all the greens, apple, and lemon. Serve chilled.

4. Beetroot Bliss

Ingredients: Beets, carrots, apples, and a hint of mint.
Instructions: Juice beets, carrots, apples, and add fresh mint. Serve over ice.

5. Berry Antioxidant Blend

Ingredients: Mixed berries (blueberries, strawberries, raspberries), spinach, and coconut water.
Instructions: Blend all ingredients until smooth.

6. Carrot-Orange Energizer

Ingredients: Carrots, oranges, and turmeric.
Instructions: Juice carrots and oranges, add a pinch of turmeric, and serve.

7. Pineapple-Mango Delight

Ingredients: Pineapple, mango, banana, and coconut milk.
Instructions: Blend fruits with coconut milk until smooth.

8. Cucumber-Mint Refresher

Ingredients: Cucumber, mint, lime, and green apple.
Instructions: Juice cucumber, mint, lime, and apple. Serve over ice.

9. Ginger-Lemon Zinger

Ingredients: Ginger, lemon, apples, and spinach.
Instructions: Juice ginger, lemon, apples, and spinach. Enjoy chilled.

10. Turmeric Golden Juice

Ingredients: Turmeric root, carrots, oranges, and pineapple.
Instructions: Juice turmeric, carrots, oranges, and pineapple. Serve over ice.

11. Blueberry Brain Boost Smoothie

Ingredients: Blueberries, bananas, Greek yogurt, and almond milk.
Instructions: Blend all ingredients until creamy.

12. Avocado-Berry Bliss

Ingredients: Avocado, mixed berries, spinach, and coconut water.
Instructions: Blend until smooth for a creamy, nutritious smoothie.

13. Mango-Coconut Dream

Ingredients: Mango, coconut milk, banana, and chia seeds.
Instructions: Blend mango, coconut milk, banana, and add chia seeds. Blend until smooth.

14. Peachy Keen Smoothie

Ingredients: Peaches, plain yogurt, almond milk, and a dash of cinnamon.

Instructions: Blend all ingredients until creamy.

15. Green Tea Infusion

Ingredients: Green tea, pineapple, kale, and honey.
Instructions: Brew green tea, let it cool, and blend with pineapple, kale, and honey.

16. Strawberry-Kiwi Energizer

Ingredients: Strawberries, kiwi, spinach, and orange juice.
Instructions: Blend all ingredients until smooth.

17. Cherry Almond Bliss

Ingredients: Cherries, almond butter, Greek yogurt, and almond milk.
Instructions: Blend until creamy and enjoy the nutty-cherry goodness.

18. Banana Walnut Smoothie

Ingredients: Banana, walnuts, dates, and milk.

Instructions: Blend banana, walnuts, dates, and milk for a delightful smoothie.

19. Melon Mint Refresher

Ingredients: Cantaloupe, honeydew, mint, and coconut water.

Instructions: Blend melons with mint and coconut water for a refreshing treat.

20. Cocoa-Berry Delight

Ingredients: Mixed berries, cocoa powder, banana, and almond milk.

Instructions: Blend berries, cocoa powder, banana, and almond milk for a chocolatey delight.

Conclusion

In the culinary journey through the pages of the "Dementia Cookbook for Seniors," we've embraced the power of nourishing both body and mind. These recipes aren't just about ingredients; they're a symphony of flavors designed to ignite memories, soothe the soul, and support cognitive well-being.

As we close this chapter, let the kitchen become a haven of joy, connection, and resilience. May each dish spark not just taste but a sense of vitality, creating moments of comfort and delight in the face of challenges.

This cookbook isn't merely a guide; it's a tribute to the enduring spirit and the simple yet profound pleasure found in every nourishing bite. Let the heart of the kitchen continue to beat, echoing the shared stories, laughter, and love that make every meal a celebration of life.